"Dr. Saul's *Conscious Parenting* offers a brief, down-to-earth approach to the complexities of parenting in the 21st century. By defining the Parental Awareness Threshold, Dr. Saul is encouraging adults to be mindful of the goals that we all hold dear for our children, and he is reminding us to be purposeful in all of the interactions that we have with our children. Although implementing this approach demands a willingness to pause, reflect, adapt, and perhaps even apologize, *Conscious Parenting* teaches us how to develop the safe, stable, and nurturing relationships that build the healthy children of today, the responsible citizens of tomorrow, and the engaged, conscious parents of the next generation."

—ANDREW GARNER, MD, PHD, Clinical Professor of Pediatrics, Case Western Reserve University School of Medicine

"Remember these three words: Parental Awareness Threshold. They are your guide to raising better children in our post-Columbine, smartphone world. Dr. Saul continues to break new ground in *Conscious Parenting,* giving us all a roadmap to becoming better parents who will produce happier and healthier children."

—BASIL HERO, Author of *The Mission of a Lifetime: Lessons from the Men Who Went to the Moon*

"With *Conscious Parenting* and the PAT, Dr. Robert Saul offers parents more than just a tool for a better, happier life. He offers a treasure map that can help frustrated, tired mothers and fathers find their way through the seasons of raising children. Parenting isn't easy, yet most of us get more guidance and expert instruction on using our smartphones than growing new humans into adults. Bob's wisdom derives from decades as a parent—but not a perfect one, he says—and as a pediatrician. Few people I have ever met care more about children and ensuring that they have every opportunity available to them to reach their potential.

No child comes with an instruction manual. As parents we bring our personalities and even our own childhood experiences into our roles, but often we do so automatically, without examination. Becoming a conscious parent can change that. Far from a theoretical work or a medical report, this book is an accessible, usable guide that can be used by parents, grandparents, and educators to thoughtfully and deliberately interact with children, even when they test every ounce of our patience. It is indispensable for community programs and workshop leaders who are reaching at-risk families or simply those who want to do better than the generation before. The goal is simple. The work is difficult. But this short book can help guide the way."

—CHRIS WORTHY, Writer

"As a parent, I think back on my worst moments, and inevitably they are the ones when I was in conflict with my children. Things were going down the tubes, we were both upset, and no one went to bed happy. What if there was a way to replace all of these moments with episodes of loving kindness, when we understand what our children need and respond appropriately? Pediatrician, father, and author Dr. Robert Saul now adds to his estimable body of work *Conscious Parenting*, a book that offers solutions to the hardest moments in parenting by helping us become more aware caregivers. Introducing the concept of the Parental Awareness Threshold, Dr. Saul synthesizes the newest and most exciting developments in psychology, philosophy, and mindfulness to offer parents a system that will help them cope with the most challenging moments that child-rearing has to offer, an opportunity to turn tears into hugs and children into warm, caring adults."

—DAVID L. HILL, MD, Pediatrician and
Author of *Dad to Dad: Parenting Like a Pro*

"Bob Saul continues his advocacy for children with a thoughtful approach to parenting in his new book, *Conscious Parenting*. As an educator for 45 years, I have seen the results of good and less-than-good parenting. This book provides the tools for those who want to be good parents. We need to create a short course for parents to help them lead their children to be healthy, happy and productive adults with *Conscious Parenting* as the textbook. Thank you, Dr. Saul, for your passionate advocacy for children."

—RAY L. WILSON, JR., PHD, Retired Educator

"Much of what influences children and youth does not occur in a classroom, but at home. Indeed, the success of our K-12 educators depends on knowledgeable and caring parents who are aware of and address their children's physical, emotional, and academic needs. Few people have a clearer understanding of this than Dr. Robert Saul. In *Conscious Parenting*, Dr. Saul—drawing on his previous scholarship and decades of experience as a pediatrician—offers both timely information and effective strategies that parents can use to build healthy and meaningful relationships with their children, especially during this hyper-competitive and highly stressful era in which we find ourselves. It is not an exaggeration to say that teachers could have a much greater impact on their students if more parents would implement Dr. Saul's recommendations. Anybody who cares about the people who will shape our future should read this book!"

—A. SCOTT HENDERSON, PHD, Professor of Education, Furman University

"Parenting is perhaps both the most important and most difficult challenge we face as adults. Dr. Saul's years of practical experience in providing parenting guidance provide a platform for the ideas he presents here. Relationships are critical to being a successful parent. Relationships that are developmentally appropriate to the needs of the child, relationships between both parents and the rest of the family and relationships between the family and the community provide a framework for promoting optimal health and development. Dr. Saul provides a guide to parenting that encompasses a conscious awareness of the vital importance of these connections."

> **—FRANCIS E. RUSHTON, MD**,
> Pediatrician and Author of *Family Support in Community Pediatrics: Confronting the Challenge*

"Bob Saul has been involved with parenting directly and in his lengthy and passionate work as a pediatrician with children and families over time. This book offers direct and relevant guidance to parents in this exciting and at times difficult journey."

> **—JAMES M. PERRIN, MD**, Professor of Pediatrics, Harvard Medical School, John C. Robinson Distinguished Chair in Pediatrics, MassGeneral Hospital for Children

"Dr. Saul's *Conscious Parenting* book provides an extremely valuable tool for the parenting journey. Building on his lifetime of pediatric experience and his previous books, he continues to be a valued advocate for children and parents everywhere."

—ROBIN LACROIX, MD, Professor of Pediatrics, University of South Carolina School of Medicine, Greenville, Chair, Department of Pediatrics, Prisma Health Children's Hospital-Upstate

"Advice that every parent can use and embrace. Dr. Saul teaches us that parenting is hard but can be mastered with practice and insight. In the hyper-competitive world of contemporary American parenting, Dr. Saul's advice in *Conscious Parenting* is a breath of fresh air that every family will benefit from reading."

—PAUL SMOLEN, MD, Pediatrician and Author of *Great Kids Don't Just Happen* and *Can Doesn't Mean Should*

"In his latest book, *Conscious Parenting: Using the Parental Awareness Threshold*, Dr. Robert Saul offers families a way to incorporate adult self-reflection and age-suitable parenting strategies. His suggestion that parents take the time to identify their own feelings when faced with a parenting dilemma leads to greater awareness of the child's perspective as well. Filled with examples from birth through the teen years, this book includes valuable tools for supporting families as they find a path to resolve conflicts in ways that support children's autonomy and build positive adult/child relationships. The ultimate goal, of course, is to help parents and others in raising caring and responsible citizens."

—ROBERTA L. SCHOMBURG, PHD,
Executive Director, Fred Rogers Center for
Early Learning and Children's Media

"Dr. Robert Saul's *Conscious Parenting* (PAT) is not so much a book about what to do when your child screams, hits, lies, or sulk, but a guide for how to THINK about what to do; how to assess your immediate emotional reaction, and how to consider the optimal response. His simple and clear framework of Parent Awareness Threshold will help parents be more thoughtful, in-tune with their children's needs and motivations, and aware of their own triggers and knee-jerk reactions. The PAT model is deceptively simple and Dr. Saul illustrates in concrete ways how to apply it. But the task of conscious (and conscientious) parenting is formidable. This book can be a mentor and companion for this most important challenge."

—RACHEL BIALE, MSW, author of *What Now? 2-Minute Tips for Solving common Parenting Challenges*

To parents and caregivers everywhere
We all need a map!

Conscious Parenting:
Using the Parental Awareness Threshold

by Robert A. Saul, MD

Published by

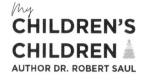
CHILDREN'S CHILDREN
AUTHOR DR. ROBERT SAUL

www.mychildrenschildren.com

CONSCIOUS PARENTING

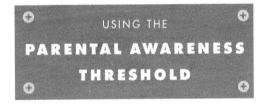

USING THE

PARENTAL AWARENESS THRESHOLD

ROBERT A. SAUL, MD

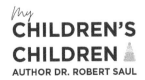

My
**CHILDREN'S
CHILDREN**
AUTHOR DR. ROBERT SAUL

TABLE OF CONTENTS

Foreword

There is no more precious resource on this earth than our children. They represent our future. All of us have been children, but not all of us have been parents, which brings with it its own sacred responsibility. Parenting—a roadmap to good parenting—is what Dr. Robert Saul gives us here in his third book on what it takes to raise healthy and productive children who can go on to contribute to the common good of society.

There is no one right way to raise children, but there are identifiably wrong ways to do so, and in *Conscious Parenting* Dr. Saul offers us a measurable method for parenting: the PAT (Parental Awareness Threshold). PAT will resonate for any parent who has struggled in the very trying times in which we live. According to a report published in 2019 by the *Journal of the American Medical Association,* teen suicides and rates of anxiety and depression are at an all-time high. I observed this firsthand in my time as executive director of Positive Directions, The Center for Prevention and Counseling. The past decade left me and our staff of seasoned psychologists looking for new ways to give parents and their children new tools for managing the anxiety and depression which is crippling so many of our young people today.

Incredibly, the stress kids face today begins in kindergarten and continues right through high school as they come under pressure to get into the so-called "right college." The focus is on test scores, good grades, and chasing the right extracurricular activities to round out one's college application. What's missing in all of this is something rarely emphasized in America's educational system, the foundation for what Aristotle believed are the two virtues vital for creating a healthy society: devotion to something greater than oneself, and the pursuit of what he called *the common good*. For democracy to work effectively, it is necessary to instill, not just in our youth, but in everyone, the notion that we're not just living for ourselves, but that we live for the community.

As you will discover from Dr. Saul, community and civic participation can have immeasurable mental health benefits for our children. You will also learn about the five steps to community improvement: 1) learn to be the best parent you can be, 2) get involved, 3) stay involved, 4) love for others, 5) forgiveness. Of equal importance is to give one's children responsibility at a young age. Children need to learn from their mistakes and how to move on from them. If you rob them from experiential learning, they will never come into their own.

Much of what you read in this pioneering book is logical, evidence-based, and in many instances counterintuitive to today's conventional wisdom about child-rearing and good parenting. We need to reconfigure our parenting skills and educational system so that it emphasizes more community involvement. The focus on the self leads to self-absorption, which ultimately can lead to unhealthy behaviors—as we are learning from school psychologists around the country. Fortunately, there is another path that we can follow to lasting success, and the Parental Awareness Threshold is the prescription to get us there.

—**BASIL HERO**, Author, *The Mission of a Lifetime: Lessons From the Men Who Went to the Moon*

Does anybody have a map?
Anybody maybe happen to know how the hell to do this?
I dunno if you can tell
But this is me just pretending to know

So where's the map?
I need a clue
'Cause I'm flying blind
And making this up as I go.

"Anybody Have a Map?" Lyrics by Benj Pasek and Justin Paul

(From *Dear Evan Hansen,* Broadway musical)

Introduction

Parenting is sometimes considered an innate process—as if everything is straightforward and will easily fall into place over the years from birth to adulthood. Conceiving children does not properly prepare us for the nurturing, physical and emotional, needed to raise healthy children.

An innate ability implies that we are born with the ability and we just need to "untap" it at the right time with just the right amount of emotional energy. And that it will be obvious how to use this ability at each juncture in our parenting journey.

In my opinion, nothing could be farther from the truth. Parenting in today's society is complex. There are so many factors tied to parenting. Parenting requires instruction from multiple places, assistance from a variety of resources and constant tinkering as we learn what we did right and what we need to improve. This book will provide a basic framework, a map, for such a process.

As the quote from *Dear Evan Hansen* above so aptly notes, we really do need a map to help guide our parenting journey. We are now two decades into the twenty-first century. Have the principles of parenting changed? Are there "new" principles that can be brought forth? I contend that the principles have not changed (to raise our children to be capable adults, i.e. engaged citizens), but the methods have evolved. In today's society, with its digital bombardment (TV, music, smartphones, computers, tablets, etc.), it is too easy to get out of touch with the basics of parenting.

Parenting challenges vary over the life of the child and often overlap with the lives of multiple children (sibs) in the family. Families might be confronted with multiple issues simultaneously.

- How do you deal with feeding an irritable infant when you are a tired, exhausted parent and you are trying to decide if you need to take the car keys away from your teenager?

- How do you have the strength to send your five-year-old to kindergarten when she is crying all the way to the school?

- How do you protect your children from the threat of bullying and ensure that your children will not be bullies?

- How do you control the exposure to potential substance abuse in your teens while dealing with problems at work that threaten your financial well-being?

How do we do these things? Well, the Parental Awareness Threshold (PAT) is a valuable tool and can help! The PAT can

- Help you sort out the multiple issues with an irritable infant, an exhausted parent and a defiant teenager.

- Help you find the strength to take a distressed child to school.

- Help you deal with the various facets of bullying.

- Help you navigate the risk of teenage substance abuse while dealing with personal issues at work.

The PAT guides parents in a logical way to analyze their current situation (their emotional state in a given situation) with regard to the threshold and then take actions consistent with a three-step process to pause, assess and choose the path forward in the context of a loving parent.

A quick example—a four-year-old refuses to eat their vegetables at dinner. "What should I do?" a parent will ask. The PAT will guide the parent to determine their emotional status ("Why am I arguing with my child about food? What is the best way to deal with this situation?") and then pause ("Ok, take a deep breath"), assess ("Remember, this child is only four years of age and doesn't understand why I consider vegetables to be so important") and choose ("Ok, how can we resolve this without raising our voices and causing emotional distress?"). We all know that relatively small things can quickly escalate to major conflicts that should be avoided. Parents using the PAT will have the tools to deal with such situations and seek reasonable solutions. It is never easy, and that is why parenting tools, like conscious awareness and the PAT, can provide significant help.

In the chapters that follow, this book will suggest *conscious awareness* as a way forward and provide a vital tool, the PAT, to deal with multiple challenges one at a time and potentially simultaneously.

Simply put, parenting in the twenty-first century requires a **conscious awareness of the status of the parent-child relationship.** It is the learned ability, not the innate ability, of parents to understand their interactions with their children and to change (adjust like a stereo system) their responses to maximize positive responses and minimize negative responses. Parents will find numerous suggestions on ways to enhance those opportunities, and multiple examples will be provided at various ages.

I have not been a perfect parent. I have made numerous mistakes along the way. I do not pretend be the perfect role model. I will continue to make mistakes. Such is our humanity. The ideas and concepts presented herein are those that I consider to be useful and are based on a lifetime of experience.

This lifetime of experience lends itself to a broad prospective across the almost two decades of childhood in support of conscious awareness in parenting.

Capable Adults and Good Citizens

Solidly nurtured children become good citizens as they become healthy adults, both socially and spiritually. One aspect of this book addresses parenting from the citizenship side because the only way our children and their progeny and our society can continue to improve is for all of us to have a common purpose—to care for, to love, to nurture, to empathize with, to support, and to come to the aid of others. This starts in our homes and then spreads to our community. Happiness and personal fulfillment will ensue.

An oft-stated goal of parenting is the happiness of our children. "I just want you to be happy" is a common statement for parents. Parents usually include safety (freedom from harm), good health and success (career or employment satisfaction) in that goal. With that view in mind, the happiness of our children will reflect our own success as parents and realize the dream that we have for our children. If the outcomes are as we have intended, then we will have reached our desired goal as parents.

I contend that the happiness of our children is a secondary goal and the delightful consequence of the primary goal—raising children to be good citizens via the principles of conscious parenting in the twenty-first century.

Sometimes more tangible instructions are needed for parenting. The remainder of the book will provide a series of examples and proposed solutions that can be used to maneuver the ups and downs, the hills and moguls, and the emotional roller coaster that can characterize parenting. Never straightforward and always a challenge, modern-day parenting requires help, nurturing, and encouragement. And even parents need to be doused with plenty of love. These supports serve to assist in this arduous and perpetual process called parenting.

To promote citizenship, tools will be presented to enable the development of conscious parenting skills. By the end of this manual, the qualities of a conscious parent, the instruments to use for conscious parenting (accepting instruction, active engagement and continued involvement), and the utility of the parental awareness threshold, or the PAT (with the abilities to pause at a moment of stress, to assess the situation and to choose wisely), will be discussed in detail to provide a tangible guide for all parents.

And specific examples for activity or action will be set aside in boxed text!

Ready? The PAT can serve as our map . . . so let's go!

Chapter 1

Conscious Parenting and Citizenship

P arenting is defined in many different ways. It is such an all-purpose term and used by so many folks in so many ways that it is difficult to be precise when discussing what parenting means.

The definition typically refers to the raising or rearing of a child or children, especially the care, love, and guidance given by a parent. Similarly, parenting or child-rearing can be considered the practice of promoting and supporting the physical, emotional, social, and intellectual development of a child from infancy to adulthood. For our purposes in this book, parenting also refers to the aspects of raising a child aside from the biological relationship.

Let's break it down into three main areas for purposes of discussion here—instruction, engagement and involvement.

Accepting Instruction

Aspects of Care

There are multiple parenting books that address many of the issues considered in the definitions above. Nutrition, infant care, health care, discipline, behavior, safety, and education are all critical aspects of advice that first-time parents often seek. They wish to know what their expectations should be, what changes will occur, and how they should negotiate all of these matters.

- Nutrition tends to focus on the merits of breastfeeding as the ultimate initial source of nutrition and its ongoing and lifelong effects for the benefit of children and even the mother.

> More evidence is discovered all of the time demonstrating the benefits of breastfeeding above and beyond the milk itself. The act of nurturing (holding the infant close, sharing a physical bond with milk exchange, and lovingly stroking the infant) is now known to be critical to these enhanced effects of breastfeeding.

Optimal nutrition is critical to early development as a biological need but does not guarantee excellent parenting.

- Infant care (nurturing through safe, stable relationships) is another critical component to parenting, and books promoting such are everywhere, speaking to its importance on our quest to optimize care for our children and to raise accomplished children and independent adults. Discipline and safety are the logical components of optimal infant care. Behavior is the outcome.

- Health care leading to excellent medical care is intended to maximize the physical and emotional well-being of our children. While very important, health care alone will not guarantee solid parenting.

- Education (parental and social and organized) is critical at so many levels. How parents, social influences and teachers use their influence to provide the necessary education and necessary exposure to the spoken and written word can help determine a substantial amount of the background for healthy growth.

Goal-Driven Behaviors for Instruction

An analysis of parenting often looks at specific components, not goals. I would argue that keeping the goals in mind provides a more focused approach. Goal-driven behaviors in parenting lead to specific actions and are worthy of discussion.

- Do we want our children to be capable of independence when childhood and adolescence ends and adulthood starts?

- Will this independence lead to a life of happiness?

- Will this happiness help define a successful career and fulfilling family life?

- Are these the best-defined goals for parenting?

- Who defines independence, happiness, and success?

Parenting to Raise Citizens

Previously, I advanced a paradigm that considers parenting as an exercise in raising citizens, people that take care of each other.[1] In the book *My Children's Children: Raising Young Citizens in the Age of Columbine,* the "Five Steps to Community Improvement" discussed are inherently the same steps to raise our children as citizens:

- Learn to be the best parent you can be

- Get involved

- Stay involved

- Love for others

- Forgiveness

Learning to be the best parent you can be while getting actively involved and staying involved is crucial. Yet without the empathy to exhibit love for others and exercise forgiveness in multiple ways, parenting becomes a selfish task instead of a selfless one.

> Parents can demonstrate their involvement by volunteering at schools and reading to a class. They can serve an active role at church in Sunday School. They can actively demonstrate their empathy for their fellow citizens by serving at a soup kitchen. All of these activities, and more, show their children how their parents (citizens) can care for each other every day, in and out of the home, and provide excellent role models at the same time.

We Need a Village

Parenting is not an innate ability in today's society. It requires instruction, support, work and a "village." Parents must be willing to accept the humility of nurturing their children with the help of family, friends, professionals and fellow citizens. That is what we mean by a village—all of these groups assisting with help as needed.

We should always strive to be the best parent we can be since there is always room for improvement and nobody is perfect. Learning to accept instruction and learning to interpret instruction and learning to apply this parenting instruction can be quite a struggle for young parents. It is not easy. Support from many places can be vital to success. Parents have to engage at multiple levels in the community village.

Active Engagement

Active Process

Since parenting is not a passive experience, active engagement by parents is essential.

> As noted above, parents can engage at school, church or a community organization. They can also take their children to the library and then read together instead of watching TV. They can go to the park where they can play or explore nature.

Without engagement, parenting is a one-way instead of a two-way street. Parenting should be a give-and-take exercise. With infants and younger children, parenting is a serve-and-return interaction—parents provide a stimulus, children return with a response, and the cycle continues to its logical conclusion. Children might also provide the initial stimulus while parents return the stimulus with an engaged response. The science is now clear that early brain wiring or circuitry is vitally dependent on the continuous stream of input or information that occurs with early parent-child serve-and-return exchanges. Positive exchanges lead to healthy wiring and brain connections, and negative exchanges can hamper the wiring and connections.

The same principles hold true for interaction throughout childhood and all stages of life for parents and children. Parents and children will hopefully stay engaged in a healthy and nurturing process. These interactions, when healthy, are described as safe, stable and nurturing relationships.[2]

Safe, Stable and Nurturing Relationships

Safe, stable and nurturing relationships (SSNRs) are the key to childhood wellness and eventually adult wellness. All three aspects are vital. SSNRs provide the basic framework that allow parents and children to react to stress in positive ways so that children will grow into healthy adults and parents also. Healthy adults (nurtured with SSNRs in childhood) will have fewer physical problems and are far more likely to succeed in raising healthy children that understand their responsibilities as citizens—to encourage and support all of their fellow citizens.

Continued Involvement

Forms

Parenting requires active engagement at two levels—getting involved and staying involved. Those two forms of involvement might seem the same to the casual observer. Getting involved might mean helping with after-school activities on an episodic basis, while staying involved could mean participating in sustained community activities over an extended period of time. I contend that these differences are indeed distinct and require separate emphasis.

It is mandatory for parents to get involved at so many levels. Direct involvement with their children, while intuitive or "second nature," is often lacking in a sustained way. Involvement might include the spouse or significant family support. After that, involvement extends far beyond the reaches of the residence—to schools, to faith-based organizations, and to the community. Getting involved in these spheres allows for social growth and social investment.

Social Capital

The problem with involvement is sustaining the effort beyond initial involvement. Staying involved is so important. Activities and community initiatives come and often fade for very valid reasons. Reenergizing one's efforts and staying involved demonstrates to the family and the community the commitment to make a difference and provide a positive example for the children. Robert Putnam's work *Bowling Alone: The Collapse and Revival of American Community* dramatically highlights the concept of *social capital*.[3] Social capital is the "stuff" that ties us all together—for example, goodwill, fellowship, sympathy and social intercourse.

Social capital is all of those aspects of social interaction that help us interact with our fellow citizens in meaningful ways. In a dramatic example, Robert Putnam documents how a bowling league acquaintance made the decision to donate a kidney to someone who was previously a complete stranger. The mere act of being in a bowling league (the social interaction) led to this bond. The person-to-person contact that comes with using social capital connects us all in so many ways.

Social capital is a potent community tonic that tends to enhance resolution of community problems; it can activate community resources for improvement; it can make us aware of how closely linked we all are; and it serves to improve our lives through action and interaction at so many levels.

Additional examples include working together at community food banks and being engaged citizens by voting at election time—local, state and federal.

When we accept that all of the children in our community are important and our joint responsibility, we are much more likely to ensure that all children can be involved in various recreational activities (such as soccer, basketball, baseball or others), not just our own children.

> Let's make sure that all children can sign up for community recreational activities by actively promoting the activities and actively getting them enrolled.

Twelve Powerful Words

Health care futurist Leland Kaiser has set a remarkable agenda for citizens and citizen involvement. He has suggested that for anything happening in a community, citizens should declare,

- "I am the problem"
- "I am the solution"
- "I am the resource."

Those are twelve pretty simple words, but the message is a powerful one. "I am the problem" refers to taking personal ownership of the issues in our community and acknowledging that all problems deserve our attention. "I am the solution" refers to working with our fellow citizens. "I am the resource" refers to the willingness to devote our continuing energies to the community.

So, that teenage pregnancy problem in a community is not *their* problem; it is *our* problem. The drug abuse problem present in a community is not *their* problem;

it is *our* problem. Homelessness is not *their* problem; it is *our* problem. An unacceptable school drop-out rate is not *their* problem; it is *our* problem. Only by active engagement can we truly make a difference, devoting our resources to seek joint solutions. Once we accept joint ownership in these issues, we engage as partners and recognize our joint humanity. We are now citizens, caring for each other.

Citizenship Is Our Ultimate Goal

Parents as Role Models

The goal of parenting should be to raise children to be good citizens. Parents care for their children and want the best for them. Parents are the ultimate citizen role models for their children. By exhibiting compassion, empathy and wisdom, parents nurture their children as they should their fellow citizens. Good citizens care for one another and their community—the hallmark of a democratic society. Our country is founded on such principles, and this need continues.

When parents engage positively with their fellow citizens, they do two things: 1) they help others and 2) they provide the positive example for their children. Children of all ages benefit when their parents do the right things and are willing to accept their roles as citizens dedicated to nurturing and improving the lives of others.

Happiness as a Secondary Effect

Happiness can be a secondary effect for children who are raised to be good citizens. Such children will reap the benefits of learning empathy and compassion towards their fellow citizens. They will see how working with and for one's fellow citizens can improve their own lives, their families' lives, and the lives of their fellow citizens and their communities.

> Children might be "happy" when they get that prized Christmas present, that new bike or the keys to the car for the first time. They might be "happy" when they get to watch their favorite TV show. But I would contend that real happiness will come when they realize as young adults or older adults that the ability to serve others can improve their own lives, the lives of their fellow citizens and their communities.

The discussion above (accepting instruction, active engagement and continued involvement) provides the logical prequel to a discussion about employing or including the principles of conscious awareness into parenting. The following chapter proposes ways to use those principles for effective parenting, involvement, love for others and the practice of forgiveness.

References:

1. Saul, R. A., *My Children's Children: Raising Young Citizens in the Age of Columbine.* CreateSpace Independent Publishing, 2013.

2. Garner, A., R. A. Saul, *Thinking Developmentally: Nurturing Wellness in Childhood to Promote Lifelong Health.* American Academy of Pediatrics, 2018.

3. Putnam, R. D., *Bowling Alone: The Collapse and Revival of American Community.* Touchstone Books, 2001.

Chapter 2

Conscious Parenting and Conscious Awareness

arenting in the twenty-first century requires a **conscious awareness of the status of the parent-child relationship.** Conscious awareness means that parents are committed to learning how to engage with their children in ways that enhance opportunities for success and minimize negative situations. Even negative situations can be opportunities for growth, but only if handled in the context of safe, stable and nurturing relationships (SSNRs). Negative situations (or what we sometimes think of as our failures) are incredibly powerful learning experiences and should be dealt with as opportunities for improvement and not simply as failures. This is perhaps one of the key points of conscious parenting and will be discussed in detail. Acknowledging our humanity (our ability to make mistakes) is vital to parenting and enables us to move forward.

Let's explore my definition of conscious awareness so we can further discuss how to use it for conscious parenting.

Definition

Conscious awareness is the learned ability of parents to understand their interactions with their children and to alter their responses to maximize positive responses and minimize negative responses. The specific components of this definition emphasize several things:

- <u>Learn</u>—Parents need to learn what it means to be conscious about the activities around them. They need to learn what it means to be conscious of their own feelings and actions. They need to learn what it means to be conscious of the feelings and actions of their children. This is not an innate inability in today's complex (and too often technologically burdened) society. This learning process requires work and dedication by the parents, and it is lifelong.

Parents can read the newspaper or watch balanced news stories to continually update their understanding of events. They can attend community meetings (city council or school board or parent–teacher association) to understand the issues that can be improved in the community. They can seek information from doctors and educators to understand how children respond to different stresses at different ages.

- Understand—Parents need to understand the dynamics of their interactions with their children. Only then can they be aware of the current state of the interactions (their words and actions) and their reactions to their children.

Parents can use the information learned above to understand the issues that fellow citizens and their children are dealing with. They can read books, watch educational programs, or attend classes that explain how to deal with emotions when parenting.

- Alter—The actions and reactions of parents might need to be altered to maximize positive activities and minimize negative responses. These "alterations" are similar to adjusting a stereo system to listen to music. While the music is the same, altering the volume or balance or fade controls will affect how the music is heard. Modulating adult responses is key to parenting.

> Parents can learn how to appreciate their actions and reactions to their children by having an honest observer provide feedback to the parents. That feedback provides the ability to alter adult responses.

Conscious awareness still implies a broader definition than the three components above. I explore that further below.

Key Concept

Conscious awareness implies that parents are constantly listening to their children. The concept of listening in this context means to "be present." Being present is a state of awareness that seeks to understand what is happening, to understand one's inner thoughts/emotions in the moment, to understand the emotions of those around them, and to understand their own actions and reactions and those of others around them.

Being present is an iterative process (the constant back-and-forth of human interaction, both verbal and physical). Being present recognizes that knee-jerk or dogmatic reactions are insufficient and, more often than not, will not serve to advance situations in a positive, constructive manner. Being present means that parents are in a constant state of growth and introspection. Growth and introspection help current situations and dilemmas, and future situations and their dilemmas.

When our child is talking, turn towards them, establish eye contact and actively listen. Sit up straight and do not fidget or look elsewhere. This attention to detail will serve parents well outside of the home and provide the right role model for "being present."

Critical Qualities

Each of the qualities listed below should be in the parental toolbox. They can assist in the process of being consciously aware of one's own feelings and actions. They can assist in assessing the feelings and actions of our children. They can help us in our constant assessment and reassessment of our relationships. By using these "tools," we can truly be engaged and consciously aware of our relationships and how we are doing.

All of these qualities are important, but they are broken up into two categories below—those more pertinent to citizenship and those more pertinent to parenting. These two categories essentially overlap, but it is helpful to separate them here for purposes of discussion.

> ### _Citizenship qualities_—qualities that lead
> to effective (good) citizens

- _Humility_—The act of not being arrogant and the ability to reflect a spirit of deference is so important in being honest in our relationships.

- _Sincerity_—A sincere relationship with one's loved ones requires honesty and freedom from hypocrisy. The ability to be sincere is critical to "being present" in relationships.

- _Empathy_—Parents must be able to understand the thoughts and feelings of others. Such an ability to understand what others are doing and why they are doing it allows them to put themselves into the "shoes" of others. Only then can we truly understand the actions of fellow citizens.

- _Vulnerability_—Parents often adopt a posture of dominance with their children. Yet the ability to recognize our vulnerability (and shared humanity) is necessary.

- _Love for others_—It goes without saying that love is the key element in a nurturing parental relationship. The love that parents have should be unconditional. When children exhibit inappropriate behavior, we can dislike their behavior, but we never dislike our children. The love of a parent should also be exhibited to our fellow citizens. By generously loving others, we provide the proper role model that our children need.

- *Forgiveness*—To sustain love for our children and love for others, forgiveness is absolutely necessary. Mistakes, simple and complex, will be made. Without the ability to forgive ourselves and to forgive others, we will be unable to accept these mistakes and improve the actions of our children and ourselves.

Parenting qualities—qualities that are
critical to effective parenting

- *Patience*—Patience is an incredible virtue and often difficult to manifest when childhood behavior tests us. An awareness of impatient reactions to certain situations helps us to analyze our reactions at any instant in time.

- *Persistence*—The trials and tribulations of parenthood require the ability to persist at times when it seems it would be easier to give in.

- *Optimism*—Optimism, like patience, is a vital virtue for parents. We all acknowledge that bad things will happen, yet the capacity to maintain optimism in the face of adversity can help instill a sense of hope in our children and ourselves.

- *The ability to change and the ability to not change (when necessary)*—Change is difficult, and the ability to discern when to change and when not to change is a perpetual quest in our adult lives. The same can be said about our relationships with our children—when do we alter our responses to a certain situation, and when do we stay with our set responses?

- *Sustained involvement*—There can be no quit in parenting. Parenting is of necessity ongoing. Yet sustained involvement can be taxing and oftentimes unsustainable. Creating the right balance and getting the right assistance is critical to being an aware parent.

- *Rational discourse*—The ability to engage in a meaningful dialogue by listening to others and expressing one's views in a sensible fashion without demeaning others defines rational discourse. The concept of conscious awareness applies here—*meaningful* means having an open mind; *dialogue* means an exchange of information between two people; *listening* means hearing, not talking; *expressing sensibly* means staying calm; and *without demeaning* means not placing oneself above others.

I have listed a whole smorgasbord of various traits and qualities above. Even if parents are fully engaged and employ the qualities mentioned, they need some kind of measure or gauge to judge their performance.

Before we head to the next chapter, let's review briefly the components of conscious awareness/conscious parenting presented to this point. In Table 1, we see the basics of conscious parenting (learn, understand

and alter) as presented in this chapter. Then we see the tools necessary to start the process. We will revisit these aspects in a consolidated format in Chapter 6.

In the next chapter, I will advance the concept of the Parental Awareness Threshold (PAT) as the measure by which parents should assess their actions.

TABLE 1. CONSCIOUS AWARENESS IN CONSCIOUS PARENTING

Overlying concepts—Learn, Understand, Alter

- Tools
    - **Basics**
        Accept Instruction
        Active Engagement
        Continued Involvement

    - **Qualities**

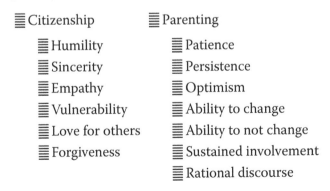

≡ Citizenship	≡ Parenting
≡ Humility	≡ Patience
≡ Sincerity	≡ Persistence
≡ Empathy	≡ Optimism
≡ Vulnerability	≡ Ability to change
≡ Love for others	≡ Ability to not change
≡ Forgiveness	≡ Sustained involvement
	≡ Rational discourse

Chapter 3

The Parental Awareness Threshold (PAT)

To properly learn the process of conscious awareness, it is helpful to consider how one application of the construct was developed. The work of Jim Dethmer and colleagues discusses the ability of conscious leaders to work with their colleagues in an effective, productive way.[1] Their work suggests that effective leaders have a significant understanding of their own actions and their interactions with others—that is, they are conscious of what they are thinking and doing in various situations.

Then, as successful leaders, they tend to be open to inquiry, curious about themselves and others and committed to learning. Those leaders that might be less successful or struggle in that role are less consciously aware of their thoughts and actions. Because of their decreased awareness, less-than-successful leaders tend to be closed in their thinking, defensive about their actions and committed to being right. And to distinguish between the two types, Dethmer and colleagues consider leaders to be either "above the line" or "below the line."

We all fluctuate in our interactions at different times, in different situations and over the course of our lives, so we will be above the line at times and below the line at times. When we are above the line, we are open, curious and committed to learning. When we are below the line, we are closed, defensive and committed to being right. We might vacillate above and below the line during specific interactions with the same people and same situations. Human nature often affects our ability to react, and yet our ability to recognize our reactions can help guide our behavior in a positive manner.

It is my contention that the concept of a line as put forth by Dethmer and colleagues can be generalized to parenting and considered as a threshold for parental awareness. The definition follows.

Definition

The Parental Awareness Threshold (PAT) is the state of conscious awareness about the past, current and future interactions of a parent with their children. It serves as a yardstick to "measure" how these interactions and their consequences occur and affect words and actions. The PAT serves to measure our degree of introspection throughout the process of parenting. This is not a magic threshold but rather one that serves to keep us aware of our inner thoughts and serves as a reminder that everything we do matters.

This threshold is analogous to the line in conscious leadership. When we are above the threshold, we are open to understanding our words and actions, we are curious about our reactions to our interactions, and we are committed to lifelong learning and improvement. When we recognize that we are below the threshold, we are closed to open dialogue, defensive in our actions and committed to being right. Let's look at some of these components:

- Open—Openness implies a willingness to be present, to listen and to accept feedback. It means that we will not jump to conclusions, especially those anchored in our biases. We will try to consider all aspects of the situation.

- Curious—Curiosity is one of the greatest parental traits. It means that we will continually explore the situation and our responses to the situation and ask ourselves how we did. We can tell ourselves "I'm just curious" as we consider how we responded and whether we could have done better.

- Committed to Learning—Living is a lifelong learning experience. We have to be committed to continually learning, improving and reflecting on our actions and the reactions of others.

Your child comes home with a report card that is not what you as a parent expect. A quick below-the-line (Below the PAT) response might be to get angry or frustrated, to yell at the child, and to quickly outline some punishment such as restricted privileges. An above-the-line (Above the PAT) response would be to calmly sit down and explore the situation and to try and understand why this occurred. The child might be defensive, so the parent will need to be open and receptive during this discussion. More information might be needed (like a discussion with the teacher). A calm and measured response might still lead to some restriction of privileges, but it can be done in the context of a loving relationship (a safe, stable nurturing relationship).

As with being below the line in a leadership role, being *Below the PAT* usually leads to unproductive interaction at any given moment and progressively over time. The PAT lends itself to a reasonable judgment of others' behavior and reasonable perception of one's own behavior.

Comparison

The comparison of the parenting PAT to the point after touchdown PAT in football is tempting to make. The PAT in football can add a point to celebrate the touchdown that was just scored. Yet the PAT in football is not guaranteed—the snap can be bobbled, the kick can be missed or it can be blocked. So, just like the football PAT, parents need to be aware that their efforts with the parental PAT will need a constant reassessment each step along the way. We might bobble our responses, we might miss our opportunity to the right thing, or our best efforts might be stymied by other circumstances beyond our control. But we keep going, knowing that we can do better the next time.

Application

Parenting is a learning experience. A parent's job is unconditional. Parents should always love their children, but they do not have to love their child's unacceptable behavior. Parents have to continually make tough decisions. Sometimes we are right, and sometimes we are wrong. Sometimes we recognize our emotions, and sometimes we are blind to our emotions. Parents supposedly know best, but when we are honest, we must acknowledge that sometimes parents are too inflexible, and sometimes parents do not live up to their promises.

By applying the PAT to everyday situations and those all-too-frequent difficult situations in parenting, parents can try to be the best parents that they can be.

In the examples starting in Chapter 5, we will look to apply the PAT at all stages of infancy, childhood and adolescence. These direct applications suggest ways to address multiple issues that parents deal with all of the time. There is no perfect solution to every situation, but the approach of conscious awareness assists parents working through all of these circumstances. It is fair to say that our parental approach and response to each will not be identical.

Individual circumstances contribute to our response. A parent's emotional state of being sad or happy or something else can certainly affect our responses. Our physical state of being well, fatigued, sick, or sleepy can also affect our responses. And the place of interaction, like at home, at a store, at church or so many other places, will affect how we react. When we analyze our response using conscious awareness, we can see that all of these factors are affecting our actions (words and deeds). We can then use all or some of the skills necessary to modulate our responses and adapt to each situation.

Incorporating the PAT into one's parenting skills models the appropriate behavior of caring citizens. Citizens should also strive to be *Above the PAT* in their interactions with each other.

Before we transition directly to the examples, let's discuss how to use the PAT in a practical way in Chapter 4.

Reference:

1. Dethmer, J., D. Chapman, K. Klemp. *The 15 Commitments of Conscious Leadership: A New Paradigm for Sustainable Success*. Dethmer, Chapman and Klemp, 2015.

Chapter 4

Above and Below the PAT (Parental Awareness Threshold)

In the previous chapter, I discussed the PAT and the state of being above or below the threshold.

Being *Below the PAT* tends to be a default position in many situations. We are typically not aware of how we show up as parents. We often just "do whatever it takes." This results in thoughts, behaviors and statements that are automatic. Decisions based on emotions tend to be *Below the PAT*. Not paying attention to how we are engaged with our children leads to missed positive opportunities as a parent. This is our challenge—how do we anticipate our responses to various conversations and situations, how do we contain our emotions, and how do we look inward as we try to be *Above the PAT* as a parent?

Let's look at what gets us from *Below the PAT* to *Above the PAT*. Shifting to *Above the PAT* requires that we set an intention, a purposeful act. We first have to know what the PAT is and what to do with it, and decide to use it. It then requires that we pause and ask ourselves, "What's happening with me right now? How am I feeling emotionally? What are the physical sensations/conditions? What are my thoughts? Where am I in relation to the PAT?"

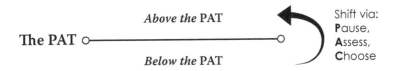

Default Position

Assessing oneself, being introspective, or holding up the mirror is easier said than done—especially in real time. Hindsight is often much better. We can review the day's events, our interactions and our parenting with a different lens. While reflection and hindsight are valuable tools, I propose that the best results are gained from being able to assess oneself *in the moment.*

Let's discuss an additional component to the Parental Awareness Threshold—a shift that is based on the ability to pause, assess, and choose wisely.

> ### *IN REAL TIME*
>
> Your child spills a drink in the back of the car on the way home from school. You are frustrated and upset that they spilled the drink after you told them to be careful. You yell at them and then pull over to clean up the mess. During the cleanup, you find out that their book bag shifted during the car ride and knocked the drink out of their hand. Now you feel badly that you overreacted.

PAUSE

In order to pause, a certain amount of knowledge is required, followed by buy-in, and followed then by practice—lots of practice, and daily practice with reminders to practice. Athletes repeatedly practice certain skills to excel. Parents need to do the same. In order to form new neural pathways in the brain, dedication and repeated practice of these skills are needed.

Our default reactions tend to come from simpler times when we merely reacted to things in the environment. As a result of a stimulus, we quickly jump to what we "know," which is often hardwired and requires the least amount of cerebral effort. This is natural, normal human behavior.

Being aware of this pattern helps us understand it. Understanding leads to becoming more familiar and comfortable. Being more familiar makes it less threatening to explore our behavior further and to adopt curiosity around how we respond to stimuli. Once we have this tackled, we must embrace these ideas as a legitimate pathway towards growth and thereby set our intention to explore further. At this stage, we buy into the idea that being present really matters. Pausing really matters; it makes the difference between *reacting* and *responding*.

IN REAL TIME

In the example above, the PAUSE might have involved taking a deep breath, pulling over, and then starting the cleanup. During the cleanup, there could have been a discussion about the circumstances that led to the spill. Our immediate frustration with the spill might have been toned down, and our assumption that our child was not being careful would have been proven wrong. We would have reacted less and responded more.

We need to practice stopping and looking inward. This has not yet been hardwired into our being. The more practice, the more hardwired it can become.

ASSESS

An honest assessment of oneself is difficult at best. We have a strong tendency towards biases. For most of us, we assess ourselves either too harshly or too leniently. This depends upon your background, upbringing, socialization and all the history you carry. If your inner voice is one of *criticism*, you might be harsh in your assessment. If your inner voice is one of *praise*, you might assess your behaviors more favorably.

Having the ability to get feedback on our own behavior is extremely helpful. We often don't see ourselves as others see us. We get wrapped up in our own "stuff" and cannot see the forest through the trees.

IN REAL TIME

In the example above, the ASSESSMENT might have been to honestly note that we assumed that our child wasn't paying attention and wasn't being careful as instructed. This assessment might still be right but can only be proven after careful review of the situation. Self-assessment of one's assumptions or biases can be quite helpful, yet it is very tough to do on a consistent basis.

Establishing a "learning partner" is an ideal way to manage this challenge. A learning partner is another individual with whom you have a trusted relationship. The use of honesty and candor in giving and receiving feedback is critical to this process. The learning partner will be authentic, open, curious, and have the ability to be objective (or more objective) about your behavior. All feedback is given and received with grace and love, in the spirit of helping to learn and grow. And you can have more than one learning partner.

An example of a learning partner could be the parent's sibling. The parent could approach their brother or sister and discuss with them their actions and reactions to certain situations. The trusted sibling can then offer an honest assessment, agreeing with their responses or offering another view that is not embedded in the emotion of the moment. Separated from the situation and all of the emotion, the trusted sibling can assist the parent by assessing the parent's ability to PAUSE, ASSESS, and CHOOSE.

Trusted friends can also be learning partners so long as the parent accepts that the response from the trusted friend will hopefully be honest and might be difficult to accept. Parents can serve as learning partners for one another, as long as it is understood that each has some skin in the game. It may be harder to be objective if they share a child.

Yet many parents do not have learning partners. They need to be able to practice their own introspection and self-assessment. This is quite difficult. For parents in this situation, some additional resources are listed at the end of the book.

Feedback is great. It's a chance to learn something. It's a practice in being open and curious about what another person has to say or what your own inner self has to say. However, feedback can also be inaccurate, subjective, or it might just "not fit." The receiver has the option to take the feedback, digest it, process it, reflect upon it and then use it (or not).

CHOOSE

If you have practiced pausing (a lot) and have found a trusted learning partner with whom you've exchanged feedback (a lot), considering and making a choice is much easier. Making a choice may mean taking a risk by being open, vulnerable and perhaps trying something different or new. Once you have let your guard down with a learning partner or your own inner voice, it provides a pathway to making different choices and taking other risks.

IN REAL TIME

In the example above, the CHOICE would have been to take that deep breath and choose to respond calmly without flying off the handle and assuming the worst. That is easier said than done in the moment, yet an honest assessment of one's response might lead to a different reaction next time. And then we will have learned how to be *Above the PAT* instead of *Below the PAT*.

The choice can be very subtle. For some, the choice is to look at a situation differently, or to reframe the opinion of what's occurred. This choice isn't necessarily visible to an observer, yet it can be very profound for the individual. And it usually leads to different behavior down the road.

For others, the choice might be quite noticeable, and the behavioral change remarkable.

For instance, if a parent has self-observed or received feedback from a learning partner that he/she tends to react (or even "overreact") with an aggressive raised voice to their teenager's dirty bedroom, perhaps the choice is to lower and soften the tone of voice or consider alternative, less threatening (and likely more effective) measures.

It is important to note that the choice might be to remain the same—do the same thing in the same way as you have always done it. The choice is yours. Of course, doing things the same leads to the same results and outcomes.

Core Drivers that Impede PAT "Work"

Inherent in our human makeup is our tendency to avoid situations that pose risks to our sense of control, security, and approval. These three core drivers or wants of human behavior are deeply rooted in our brains and have served to protect us yet make it difficult to be effective in our transition from *Below the PAT* to *Above the PAT*.

• Human beings like to feel in **control**. We want to know that we have the ability to make changes and decide for ourselves. In fact, that feeling of being "out of control," lacking choices, or having no power is extremely uncomfortable to us.

- Human beings strive for **security**. We want to be secure of being OK, of having our basic needs met (physical, emotional, financial, etc.), and of the safety of our ego or our identity. When security is threatened, we become very "scarcity-minded" and begin to see things in terms of "there's not enough."

- Humans likewise are driven towards **approval**. This is the ability to be seen as adequate, part of the social fabric, and liked by others. At a primal level, humans need other humans. We want to be accepted and loved. We seek friendships, mates, and fellowships. When we lack approval, we tend to feel isolated and lonely.

- Recognizing that control, security and approval are essential components to life but can also impede our appropriate introspection and our ability to properly employ the PAT is an important step. Once we recognize those potential conflicts, we can try to make the best choices possible using the PAT model.

None of this is easy. It takes a lot of practice. Now we are ready to consider specific examples for the applications of the PAT (the Parental Awareness Threshold and Pause, Assess, Choose) in practical situations in Chapter 5.

Chapter 5

Examples for Growth and Improvement

Now that the concept of conscious parenting and the Parental Awareness Threshold (PAT) have been explored, let's look for specific examples where parents are engaged and some real-life suggestions for conscious parenting over the course of the first two decades of life.

Ages 0–1

Parenting in the first year of life, especially in the first several months, is very stressful. Parents are often fatigued, particularly first-time mothers who are breastfeeding. Parents can be bombarded from multiple fronts—family and friends. These helpful or not-so-helpful resources often present conflicting information. When parents are left to their own devices, they have to deal with situations that might be difficult to sort out.

How about a very fussy baby (perhaps colicky) and fatigued parents? Does the father just tell the mother that she can handle it because he has to get some sleep, then go to work? How does the mother handle the flood of feelings (love for her baby, the fatigue of being too busy, the fatigue from decreased sleep, the multiple emotions for which she might even question her ability to be an adequate parent, and others) yet rise to the occasion to be the nurturing, loving parent that can satisfy the needs of a fussy baby? Understanding the PAT might help!

Since the infant cannot talk, the parents must learn the signals from the infant. They must learn how to respond to basic needs (feeding, diaper changes, sleep and the like) and how to care for the infant in a loving, sustained manner that is the basis for a safe, stable and nurturing relationship (SSNR). If parents feel above the threshold (open, curious, open to learning), they can often handle the situation comfortably. If they are below the threshold (closed, defensive, resistant to learning), they will likely struggle to deal with the situation. Knowing how they are feeling can help them do what is best in this and similar situations. Knowing their feelings and where they stand regarding the PAT can help them sort out their course of actions.

In the scenario with a fussy baby, the parents should realize their own feelings ("I am tired and don't know if I can deal with this" or "My poor baby. I want to do everything I can to soothe them"). They should also realize that the infant has very limited responses (sleep, cry, eat) to early stresses. Their responses should be measured and appropriate. In this circumstance, a reasonable response might include recognizing that the baby has little control and that the parents will need to calmly deal with the fussiness and handle one issue at a time. Awareness is the key to execution, and both parents have to be a part of the plan.

This analysis might seem a bit too complex for such a straightforward situation, but I contend that learning one's PAT in this scenario is critical in order to handle this situation well and to learn how to critically develop such skills going forward. This analysis should occur in the moment and in retrospect so the learning can be unremitting. Parenting is an ongoing process, with continuous ups and downs. This process is essential to growth as a parent.

Ages 1–2

The challenges for parents continue at every stage. As children grow they exhibit more complicated behaviors, and these behaviors are not necessarily loveable ones. In the process of exploring their world and learning what happens, children will do certain things—and the PAT might affect how parents respond.

What happens when the toddler throws their food on the floor? Like with the fussy baby in the first example, the parents' conscious awareness of their situation is critical. It could be the end of a long day and the prospect of cleaning up a mess is really annoying. Maybe the family has unrealistic expectations about toddler behavior and thinks discipline is now necessary.

It is important for parents to know "normal" behaviors and what to anticipate at each stage of life. Children are playful and love to try different things. Throwing food seems innocent to them, yet it can be quite aggravating to parents. The parents might be preparing food for the entire family and dealing with multiple issues at mealtime. Food thrown onto the floor just adds a level of annoyance the parents might not be ready for. A toddler is starting to learn limits, so parents might feel that a terse word, a shout or a pop on the hand will help teach them a lesson. All three of these responses are not appropriate in this situation.

The parent will need to take that proverbial deep breath (pause), analyze the situation (assess), and decide on the best course of the action (choose). And again, the best responses are not always the same. They can vary. But a calm, measured response is so important when dealing with a toddler. No yelling or popping should be used.

Well, this is a situation where understanding a toddler's behavior is very important, and understanding a parent's response using the PAT will be critical to a measured reaction to throwing food. Being *Above the PAT* (being open and committed to learning normal toddler behavior) can guide parents to acceptance of different behaviors and calm responses to those behaviors.

Ages 2–5

At this age range, children are really learning how their behavior can affect the behavior of others. They learn that their actions, more often than not, lead to a significant reaction in the adults around them. They learn their behaviors will change the behavior of the adults and allow them to get what they want.

At this age, there is generally some discussion about the use of discipline for dealing with undesirable behavior. Remember that the root word for discipline is "disciple" and that disciples teach. Discipline should therefore be a learning experience, not a punishment experience. Parents need to use conscious awareness and the PAT to provide positive discipline their children. They need to take that deep breath (pause), analyze the situation (Am I *Below the PAT* or *Above the PAT*?) and choose a more positive approach to correct the behavior. In that way, discipline becomes positive rather than serving as a negative punishment.

How should I handle temper tantrums? Temper tantrums are a normal developmental stage. Temper tantrums in children are an example of behavior that is meant to change the behavior of the parents. The parents are the "audience," and the children expect for their parents to respond and give in to their wants/desires.

> The PAT in this circumstance should guide the parent to be aware of this behavior. Two responses are most appropriate—1) ignoring the behavior and 2) letting the tantrum run its course. Both of these require the PAT (knowing what to expect and how to deal with it calmly) to understand the dynamic at play and to not get caught up in the raw emotions of the moment.

If the parents are *Below the PAT* (defensive and committed to being right) and not aware of the "childish" behavior, they will likely get embroiled in this situation and respond in a similar manner by yelling or screaming. By being *Above the PAT* and knowing what to expect and how to respond to temper tantrums, parents can endure temper tantrums and watch them diminish in frequency and intensity. Equally important is learning the ability to identify the triggers that might lead to tantrums.

Such triggers might include fatigue, hunger or a new social setting. The discomfort that the child might feel in these situations can certainly predispose the child to try to get out of the situation by a tantrum. By identifying these triggers, parents learn how to be proactive and avoid certain situations.

As previously mentioned, parents should try to analyze their responses in the moment (in real time) and in retrospect so that their learning can continue.

What should I do when my child runs away from me? Children at this age are exploring the limits of their freedom. It is not unusual for a child, sometimes playfully, to bolt from their parents and run into a potentially dangerous situation. The circumstances need to be handled quickly to avoid harm, but they should always be handled in a loving manner. This can be very difficult, especially when parents are in a panic mode. They can be both worried about their child's well-being and angry at the child's actions. The child's disobedience can make it very difficult to have a sense of awareness about the PAT.

In the moment, immediate corrective actions are needed. But after the situation has been defused, parents need to be sure that their response was measured. A retrospective (after-the-fact) review of the response and its relationship to the PAT is always helpful since the situation might arise again.

Responses *Below the PAT* (anger or raised voices) can certainly occur in such a situation. Recognizing one's relation to the PAT and attempting to improve it for future interactions is crucial for conscious awareness in parenting.

What should I do when my child strikes me during a temper tantrum? During a temper tantrum, it is not unusual for a child to flail their arms and legs. Whether intentional or unintentional, the child might strike the parent. Whether the parent is just startled or the parent is hurt, a parental reaction might be to strike back at the child. Responding with physical punishment is not appropriate.

It is very difficult to keep one's composure and even consider your relationship to the PAT in such a situation. As in the example of the child running away from parents, a measured response to being hit by a young child (such as calmly noting that the behavior was not acceptable) is important, and then an honest assessment of the response after the fact is critical to continued improvement as a parent. Did we overreact or handle the problem calmly? Were we able to keep a soft voice and explain why hitting people is not right? If we acted too impulsively, did we apologize and explain our mistakes?

We all respond inappropriately at times. This is human nature. But the ability to assess our relationship to the PAT (above or below the threshold) will serve to help us in our parenting now and in continued interactions. The equilibrium of life (being *Above the PAT* or *Below the PAT*) will always be in a state of flux due to our humanity. Improving our parenting through conscious awareness can help in the perpetual cycle of parenting.

Ages 5–10

Children in this age range understand more and more things about the consequences of their behavior but still have immature responses to various situations. Parents are likewise challenged by the roller coaster of their children's actions and their own variable reactions to their children. The PAT is a crucial yardstick for parenting in this age group.

Your child does not want to go to school. How should you react? School anxiety is not an uncommon problem in childhood. Parents need to try to understand all of the dynamic factors at play—the situation at school, the academic challenge for the child, the emotional well-being of the child, the family situation and more. So many aspects of the situation might contribute to school refusal. Given all of the possibilities, parents need to seriously consider everything in mounting a response. There is no set response to handling school anxiety.

While providing a safe, stable nurturing relationship, parents can now analyze the situation and consider the best way to assist their child. Assessment questions to ponder include

- Are there some simple measures that will help?

- Are there other issues that also need to be addressed?

- Can I simply accompany my child to the classroom for several days and the problem will be resolved?

- Who do I need to involve to help deal with this issue?

In addition to looking for external causes and external assistance, parents should use the PAT to evaluate their view of the situation and how they can pause, assess and maybe choose a method to help their child. Using the principles discussed in Chapter 2, parents can engage in the perceived best plan and adapt their responses appropriately.

What happens when my child won't go to bed on time or bedtime is a struggle every night? Bedtime can be battle time in some households. It is imperative for parents to avoid battles where possible. Using the PAT, parents can think ahead and plan activities and a strategy leading up to bedtime that will avoid a struggle. Sometimes it is easy to know what to do but difficult to actually do it. Parents might be aware of an impending difficulty and know how to avoid it. But at the end of the day, everyone is tired. Parents are tired and children are often exhausted. And when people are tired, emotions tend to be raw and reactions exhibit "frayed nerves."

In this scenario, parents need to take a step back—they need to pause (often hard to do when fatigue sets in); they need to assess the situation (What are we doing right? What can we do better? How can we remove the "drama" from the situation?); and then they need to choose a plan, perhaps taking a risk, that will lead to a better outcome and a mutually satisfying end of the day. The parents need to establish a better post-dinner/pre-bedtime schedule that will lead to a more likely positive outcome.

Knowing one's relation to the PAT (hopefully shifting from *Below the PAT* to *Above the PAT*) is critical to a positive outcome. There will be successes and failures in this process, but the goal is to have more successes than failures over time and the eventual strengthening of the child-parent bond in the context of a safe, stable and nurturing relationship.

My children fight like "cats and dogs." How do I stop that? Siblings are often involved in disagreements. A lot of those seem to be inevitable, what with the conflicting interests of children. Given that, parents need to assess any given situation and anticipate potential conflicts.

By anticipating conflict, parents are **Above the PAT** because they are curious, open and committed to learning how to deal with difficult situations. If they are closed and defensive (**Below the PAT**), they are more likely to respond with frustration instead of measured patience. But parents have the opportunity to be more proactive when it comes to sibling conflict. Parents learn by experience what triggers are likely to lead to a sibling argument. When those triggers are present, parents need to change the situation or engage in a distracting behavior. Sibling conflicts can often be averted and family discord minimized.

Ages 10–20

The second decade of life tends to be a tumultuous time. Pre-teens and teenagers acquire more knowledge and worldly experiences. Along with that, they have greater expectations of being able to influence others. Yet their brains are not fully developed, and their level of maturation varies widely. There is currently good evidence to suggest that brain development is not really done until the mid-twenties. Given that, parents can expect to be in for a "rough ride" and definitely be open, curious and committed to learning. The shifts in behavior and emotions in this age group require compassionate, loving parents who are measured in their responses. These measured responses can try our patience and definitely require an acute understanding of the parental PAT.

My child's grades are not good and their school performance is falling off. A quick parental response might be frustration followed by a stern warning and restriction of privileges. It is important to take a step back (pause) and see what is happening (assess).

> There are so many factors that might contribute to poor school performance. Are there learning disabilities? Are there academic challenges? Are there mental health problems? Is bullying a factor? Are there peer relation problems? Are there family problems? This list could go on and on. The point is that it is incumbent on the parents to try to understand the situation and then choose an appropriate plan of action. They need to try to take the emotion out of the decision.

Emotional decisions tend to be *Below the PAT*. A calm, measured decision done *Above the PAT* is more likely to be helpful to a long-term solution. From the old expression "Rome wasn't built in a day," we can also note that problems are not corrected overnight. The process occurs over time in the context of a loving supportive relationship (i.e., a safe, stable and nurturing relationship).

My teenager stays up too late. How do I get her to go to bed? It is not unreasonable for parents to set sensible rules in the house. Electronic devices should be turned off after a certain time. Homework should be completed by a certain time.

Even in the teen years, there should be a set time for bed. Why? We know that sleep is a critical element in health, both physical and mental. So sleep times are important not because "I said so" but because "I love you and want what is best for your health." The latter sentence takes an *Above the PAT* instead of a *Below the PAT* approach. Being calm and offering a reasoned approach, even when the teenager is not calm and reasoned, is so important and demonstrates the correct behavior. Parents must model good behavior for their children if their children are to eventually learn rational behavior.

Remember that individual teenage "battles" are not won or lost. Parenting in the teen years is a process with ups and downs. And parents need to be in it for the long haul.

I am worried that my child is using drugs or alcohol. A critical part of the Parental Awareness Threshold is awareness of the child's well-being. It is naïve to think that parents can know everything about all aspects of their teenager's life. Teens have a fair degree of autonomy and can engage in a variety of activities, both good and bad.

Parents must have an awareness that all children can succumb to temptations. It is not *Below the PAT* to think such thoughts. I contend that such considerations are actually healthy, *Above the PAT*, by being concerned about unhealthy influences for teens. Further, it is appropriate to question our youths in a healthy, loving way. Appropriate measures to consider include concern for the teen's mental health, questioning of activities and establishing a trusting relationship to allow for open, honest interactions. If a parent is concerned that a child might be using drugs, accusations could be counterproductive.

Open lines of communication are crucial to support the teen, the family and the parent. All three (child, family unit and parent) are important going forward. An understanding of school performance, peer relationships and after-school activities is also very important.

My child is too anxious or seems depressed at times. It is crucial to know the mental health of your children. Now, that statement might sound naïve. It is hard to know what is going on in someone's head, but their actions can speak volumes about their mental status.

Changes in sleeping patterns, grades, behaviors or friendships can provide valuable clues about the need for potential intervention by the parents. Anxiety or depression or combinations of both are certainly signals that parents need to have an honest discussion with their teenagers.

A safe, stable and nurturing relationship with your teen and being *Above the PAT* will help. Yet often teens in distress have a tough time with sharing their concerns. Choosing awareness (*Above the PAT*) is so important; parents are a vital source of help. Counselors or mental health professionals are often needed, but open communication in the family will greatly facilitate sharing. As stated above, the swings in emotions and behavior (which can be relatively "normal") need to be evaluated in a broad context and dealt with as calmly as possible. Failure to act can have serious short-term and long-term consequences.

How do I know that my child is a responsible driver? Parents have to know that their children are responsible drivers. With the keys to a car, teenagers are now in charge of a potentially lethal instrument—and teens are the drivers with the greatest accident rate.

Due diligence by the parents, with appropriate expectations for driving (obey the rules of road, no speeding, no texting and driving), must occur. Driving is a privilege, not a right, which demands close attention to the matters at hand. Restriction of driving privileges should be used as needed.

Parents are in charge of their teen drivers. They can still be *Above the PAT* (by using praise when it is appropriate and by anticipating potential problems yet dispassionately engaging in the necessary conversation) and exert the necessary control over this important activity.

So many children have problems controlling their weight. How can I make sure that they eat healthy and don't get overweight? This problem is an issue for everyone in our country. By and large, we all eat too much. And we know the consequences of that—obesity.

> Parents need to set the example by eating healthy, restricting the availability of junk food and saying the right things. This latter point is so important. Teens should not be shamed into submission. They should not be told that they are "fat" or otherwise bullied.

"Fat shaming" does not lead to effective change and is *Below the PAT*. The American Academy of Pediatrics has emphasized a useful tool to encourage healthy eating and ways to reduce weight.

> The 5-2-1-0 paradigm has been suggested—eat 5 fruits or vegetables a day, have no more that 2 hours of non-homework related screen time (TV, tablet, smartphone), have 1 hour of exercise per day, and drink 0 (zero) sugary-sweetened beverages. These changes have been shown to be effective.

Such a paradigm uses *Above the PAT* techniques: proactive interventions that are delivered in a caring, loving relationship. Shaming our children about their body and how they look (being *Below the PAT*) can have negative consequences. Often when children are subjected to a barrage of belittling comments, their behavior might lead to an eating disorder with inadequate nutrition. The take-home message here is that parents and children need to work together in an environment that encourages honest yet loving exchanges that allow for both to pause, assess, then choose wisely as they work together for their mutual benefit.

Chapter 6

The Path Forward

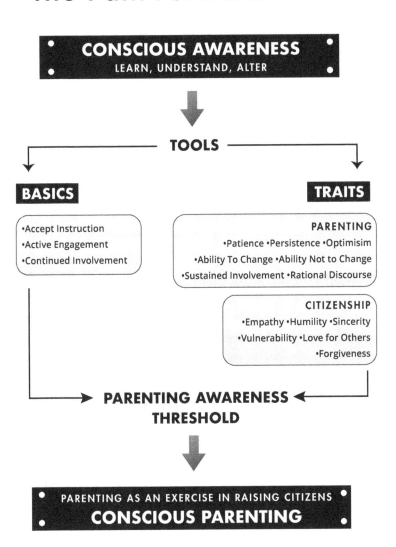

CONSCIOUS AWARENESS
LEARN, UNDERSTAND, ALTER

TOOLS

BASICS
- Accept Instruction
- Active Engagement
- Continued Involvement

TRAITS

PARENTING
- Patience •Persistence •Optimisim
- Ability To Change •Ability Not to Change
- Sustained Involvement •Rational Discourse

CITIZENSHIP
- Empathy •Humility •Sincerity
- Vulnerability •Love for Others
- Forgiveness

PARENTING AWARENESS THRESHOLD

PARENTING AS AN EXERCISE IN RAISING CITIZENS
CONSCIOUS PARENTING

Having discussed the PAT and specific examples of how to employ the PAT in real-life situations, it is worthwhile to take a step back and reflect again on the process of conscious awareness. To do so, let's review the overall concepts of conscious awareness and conscious parenting. The figure above puts all the factors into one diagram.

Conscious Awareness

The definition used herein is *the learned ability of parents to understand their interactions with their children and to alter their responses to maximize positive responses and minimize negative responses.*

Learn, Understand, Alter

I emphasized three components: 1) learn, 2) understand, and 3) alter. All three of these components are needed. Parenting and conscious awareness are learned behaviors, and parents must recognize this. They will need to understand the ever-changing dynamics of parent-child interactions. Then they will need to alter their responses to maximize positive activities and minimize negative responses. The take-home message here is to *be present* (as introduced and discussed in Chapter 2).

Tools—Basics and Traits

The basic tools are accepting instruction, active engagement, and continued involvement. The methods are divided into two broad categories of personality traits that are not mutually exclusive. Citizenship or personhood traits are empathy, humility, sincerity, vulnerability, love for others and forgiveness. Additional parenting traits include patience, persistence, optimism, ability to change, ability to not change, sustained involvement and rational discourse. The basic tools and traits then allow us to employ the PAT.

Parental Awareness Threshold (PAT)

As discussed in detail in Chapter 4 and then employed in Chapter 5, we can use the PAT to see how we can be *Above the PAT* more often than *Below the PAT*. By using *pause, assess* and *choose*, we take the necessary steps to be present in our interactions with our children and maximize positive interactions and minimize negative interactions. To do the latter, let's talk about the possibilities for success and areas for improvement to address. Since any possibility for success is also an area for improvement, we will discuss them together.

Raising Young Citizens

I have emphasized the importance of our children becoming good citizens, people who take care of each other. When parents engage positively with their fellow citizens, they do two things: 1) they help others, and 2) they provide the positive example for their children. They understand the "I am the problem, I am the solution, I am the resource" model of engagement. Children will benefit when parents do the right things and are willing to accept their roles in our society as citizens who nurture and improve the lives of others. It is my contention that happiness is a joyful consequence of such engagement and provides the benefit to conscious parenting.

Possibilities for Success and Areas for Improvement

1. *Are the parents right or wrong?* Conscious awareness requires a realistic assessment of the current situation. Sometimes parents are too focused on right vs. wrong and not focused enough on what makes sense in a given situation. The concept of the PAT reminds us that our default mode is, more often than not, *Below the PAT*, and it takes the conscious awareness to pause, assess and choose wisely if we are serious about getting *Above the PAT*. A thoughtful evaluation often leads to the realization

that being right or wrong isn't as important as awareness of the situation. Being right and *Above the PAT* is important, but it is possible that parents can be right about a certain situation yet be *Below the PAT*. The latter situation ("right" but *Below the PAT*) occurs when parents are dogmatic about their stance. In a life-threatening situation, such a stance is perfectly acceptable. But when parents are closed, defensive and committed to being right, negative circumstances typically occur. When parents are *Above the PAT*, they can be either right or wrong as long as they are curious, open and committed to learning. This learning hopefully leads to a successful outcome. And if it doesn't, it emphasizes an area for improvement going forward.

2. *Parents have to make tough decisions.* Tough decisions, decisions that are unpopular in the eyes of the child, are some of the most difficult moments of parenting. When our children are upset, emotions can take over and the "right" decision can seem wrong and complicate the situation. The parent's conscious awareness is crucial in this scenario. If we can calmly reflect on the various issues at hand and feel comfortable with our decision (i.e., we are *Above the PAT*), then we should stick with our choice. The key issue at play here is to be comfortable with an honest self-assessment (i.e., conscious awareness) of our actions. If we are *Above the PAT*, that is great. If

we are *Below the PAT*, then we should ask ourselves if any changes in our responses are needed. That is how we make the "right" tough decisions.

3. *Are the parents flexible or inflexible?* Much like the discussion about being right or wrong, parents can be too flexible or too inflexible when it comes to making a decision in the moment. The ability to assess one's flexibility really depends on one's conscious awareness. As we learn over the course of our parenting, we need to gain an appropriate understanding of our actions and alter our responses accordingly.

4. *Did we live up to our promises?* It is not unusual for parents to make promises to their children.

"If you behave in [fill in the situation], we will go to [fill in the treat of choice]" is a very common scenario for parents. We have all been there. But have we been faithful to our promise?

We need to be realistic about our expectations and then fulfill our promises. If we do not fulfill our promises, not only are we *Below the PAT* but also we are not as trustworthy as parents should be. Remember that safe, stable and nurturing relationships are critical for our children's wellness and lifelong health and that SSNRs are the antidote for the toxic stress that might affect children.

5. *Little things matter.* Parents tend to focus on large issues and draw the line in the sand about their decision-making. All aspects of parenting are important. Often the most incidental or inconsequential thing can have dramatic consequences in the lives of our children. What we perceive to be minor can be a major thing in the eyes of the child. So the PAT is crucial here. If we are *Above the PAT*, we are curious about how our children perceive the world. If we are *Above the PAT*, we are committed to learning what makes our children tick and how we can be a positive influence in their lives. When we are *Below the PAT*, we are closed to seeing how little things do matter and how they affect our children and our relationship with them.

6. *Parents' love is unconditional.* It is critical to always remember this. When a child's behavior becomes unacceptable, we can dislike the behavior. But we can never dislike the child. I have purposely avoided the term "hate" here. Children should always be loved even when we do not love their behavior in a given situation. Conscious awareness in parenting requires an introspective lens. The introspection of using the PAT and taking the time to pause, assess, and choose forces us to look at our relationship with our children. Are we expressing our love for our children? Have we exhibited love for our children through our actions? Have we exhibited love for others (being a positive

example and modeling appropriate behavior) in our words and actions? The PAT forces us to look inward and think about what we do.

Let's emphasize one final note about the PAT and the path forward. As previously noted, the PAT in football (point after touchdown) serves to add a point after the touchdown. It is not guaranteed. Just as the football PAT can go awry, so can a parent's attempt to use the Parental Awareness Threshold. Parents should be willing to constantly assess their actions, words and relationships as they work to make a positive difference in the lives of their children.

Chapter 7

Concluding Remarks

We have discussed throughout this book the concept of conscious parenting—parenting that emphasizes a conscious awareness of the status of the parent-child relationship. I have defined conscious awareness in this relationship as the learned ability of parents to understand their interactions with their children and to alter their responses to maximize positive responses and minimize negative responses. I firmly believe that these processes are not innate and require work and nurturing over the entire life of any parent—from the moment of conception of one's first child through the continued parenting of any children and all of their progeny. The point here is that parenting is a never-ending, lifelong learning proposition. And we all need help along the way. This book is meant to be a guide along the journey. So let's review some of the key concepts presented.

1. **Citizenship:** The goal of parenting should be to raise children to be good citizens. Good citizens care for one another and their community. Citizens that care for each other and their community are the primary components of a democratic society. The foundational bases for raising good citizens are proper instruction, active engagement, and continued involvement.

2. **Conscious Awareness:** The learned ability to understand and to alter responses as necessary can be difficult. Yet the key concept should always be kept in mind. That concept is to "be present" with active listening, seeking to understand and be in a constant state of growth and introspection. In Chapter 2, we listed numerous qualities/traits that need to be in the parental toolbox for conscious awareness to occur.

3. **Parental Awareness Threshold (PAT):** Defined as the state of understanding one's conscious awareness about the past, present and future interactions with one's children, this concept is crucial to conscious parenting. The components of openness (a willingness to be present), curiosity (continual exploration) and a commitment to learning (lifelong) define the ability to be *Above the PAT*.

4. **Above and Below the PAT:** We noted that the default "position" of human beings is usually *Below the PAT,* being closed, defensive, and committed to being right. Conscious awareness allows for us to analyze our

status and to adjust accordingly in a positive manner. Adjustments to be *Above the PAT* from being *Below the PAT* take several steps—to pause, to assess and to choose, and then engage in active practice.

In Chapter 5, we presented some examples of using conscious awareness and conscious parenting. These examples are meant to cover the various stages of childhood, but we must emphasize that each situation is unique and requires a constant assessment. Just because a situation was handled one way at one point in time doesn't mean that will be the correct way the next time.

Conscious parenting requires a review of the possibilities for success and areas for improvement that were discussed in Chapter 6. Practice, practice, practice is the key point that determines our ability to proceed on this journey called parenting.

Parenting is not innate. It requires work. There are "ups" and there are "downs" along the way. Parenting in the twenty-first century can go in the "right" direction when guided by conscious awareness and the Parental Awareness Threshold. Our success, measured in raising good citizens that care for each other and their communities, demands our constant attention and can be rewarding beyond belief. I hope the discussion herein will provide a useful guide and be satisfying for parents and children alike.

ACKNOWLEDGMENTS

This book represents my ongoing effort to use a lifetime of experience on behalf of children and families. My books—*My Children's Children: Raising Young Citizens in the Age of Columbine* (self-published in 2013), *All about Children* (illustrated children's book with Jan Yalich Betts and self-published in 2017), and *Thinking Developmentally: Nurturing Wellness in Childhood to Promote Lifelong Health* (co-authored with Dr. Andrew Garner and published by the American Academy of Pediatrics in 2018)—have led me down a path of children's advocacy and community improvement. Interested readers are invited to check out my website, www.mychildrenschildren.com, for ongoing blog entries and video postings. And it is so exciting to have so many people helping along my journey.

These efforts are always dependent on family, friends and colleagues. These folks provide counsel and advice that helped guide me. I am extremely grateful to the following for their advice, encouragement and assistance:

Blakely Amati, Lee Beers, Beth Buzogany, Paul Catalana, Lorraine Cragan-Sullivan, Kathy Crytser, Rachel Daskalov, Tony Delgado, Martha Edwards, Michelle Esquivel, Shelley Fiscus, Jane Foy, Andy Garner, Michael Gauderer, Michelle Gimmi, Jill Golden, Sally Goza, Debbie Greenhouse, Scott Henderson, Basil Hero, David Hill, Sarah Hinton, Jenny Kelley, Robin LaCroix, Julie Linton, Zac Litwack, Suzanne Manning, Crissy Maynard, Tallya McDowell, Kirby Mitchell, Tom Moran, Betty Page Ogren, Jim Perrin, Dick Riley, Francis Rushton, Martin Rutte, Janine Sally, Bill Schmidt, Roberta Schomburg, Pam Shaw, Jenn Shu, Katy Smathers, Brooke Smith, Paul Smolen, Emilie Sommer, Paul Spire, Jen Springhart, Cathy Stevens, Beth Tarini, Tracy Trotter, Kristin van Tilburg, Michael Wiederman, Nancy Wilburn, Ray Wilson, and Chris Worthy.

I am particularly indebted to Sharon Mills Wilson for her assistance with early drafts of the book and her early partnership with this effort. She was exceedingly helpful in the initial conceptualization of the conscious parenting model and the Parental Awareness Threshold.

A great deal of gratitude also goes to Jim Dethmer and his colleagues for their work in conscious leadership. I had the incredible experience to hear Jim consult with the leadership teams at my academic institution, explaining the premise of conscious leadership and the above-the-line/below-the-line concept. It is the work of

Mr. Dethmer and his colleagues that provided me the "aha!" experience to pursue this work as an extension of my other books.

Alain Park has provided invaluable editorial assistance. His comments, reviews and advice have helped sustain the necessary impetus to keep the project going forward.

The team at Koehler Books (John Koehler, publisher; Joe Coccaro, executive editor; Hannah Woodlan, associate editor; Kellie Emery, senior graphic designer) helped bring this project over the finish line with incredible skill and professionalism. They were a delight to work with.

The ultimate gratitude goes to my family. My sons, Bradley and Ben, have been the source of inspiration for all of my efforts on behalf of other children and families. And the love of my life, Jan Saul, has been there for me with constant support and encouragement for over thirty-two years now. They help provide the energy for my work, and I am forever grateful.

Bob Saul

PARENTING RESOURCES

1. Ginsburg, Kenneth R., *Building Resilience in Children and Teens: Giving Kids Roots and Wings* (3rd ed.). American Academy of Pediatrics, 2014.

2. Ginsburg, Kenneth R., *Raising Kids to Thrive: Balancing Love with Expectations and Protection with Trust*. American Academy of Pediatrics, 2015.

3. Hill, David L., *Dad to Dad: Parenting like a Pro*. American Academy of Pediatrics, 2012.

4. https://parentsasteachers.org/news/2019/5/6/this-free-program-connects-new-moms-and-dads-with-useful-tools

5. Korb, Damon, *Raising an Organized Child: 5 Steps to Boost Independence, Ease Frustration, and Promote Confidence*. American Academy of Pediatrics, 2019.

6. Kowal-Connelly, Suanne, *Parenting through Puberty: Mood Swings, Acne and Growing Pains*. American Academy of Pediatrics, 2015.

7.   Rogers, Fred, *Many Ways to Say I Love You: Wisdom for Parents and Children from Mister Rogers.* Hyperion, 2006.

8.   Rogers, Fred, *The World According to Mister Rogers: Important Things to Remember.* Hachette Books (Revised edition), 2019.

9.   Swanson, Wendy Sue, Mama Doc Medicine: Finding Calm and Confidence in Parenting, Child Health, and Work-Life Balance. American Academy of Pediatrics, 2014.

Printed in the USA
CPSIA information can be obtained
at www.ICGtesting.com
LVHW092044211123
764552LV00004B/59